FAITH

FOOD

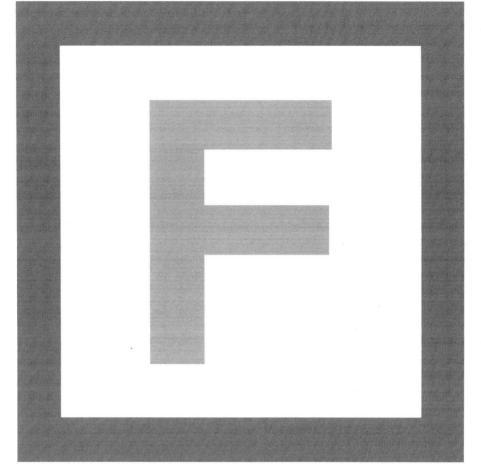

FAMILY

FITNESS

31-DAY FAITH, FAMILY, FITNESS, FOOD JOURNAL

BY BENJAMIN LEE

— INTRODUCTION —

Are you done with the EXCUSES? Are you ready for CHANGE? Then let's go! My name is Benjamin Lee. In August of 2016, I was 38 years old, fat, and without a lot of confidence. I felt like I was stuck. I wasn't happy with my weight. I wasn't happy with my body. In fact, I couldn't fit into some of my clothes. Would things ever change for me? On August 28th, 2016 things would change for me...I began my year of transformation.

I started exercising six days a week, 25-35 minutes per workout. I began eating six times per day and taking the proper supplements. And I began to do something else — I started journaling everything I did. This was a big part of my success. I planned and prepared what and when I was going to eat. I did my best to record everything I consumed. I didn't always document perfectly, but putting pen to paper helped me tremendously — it will help you too. To be intentional with your plans is powerful. Putting your thoughts down on paper is also powerful; it makes things that much more real.

I had another realization in 2016. I recognized that to transform our physical bodies we must also transform our mindset. When we get our mindset right, the body will

follow. To help get my mind right, I began to write out motivational thoughts to myself. I would write down certain phrases over and over to flood my mind with good thoughts. I also wrote my prayers out on a daily basis. I love doing this. It forces me to slow down and really think about what I'm asking and saying to God. I also began to make a gratitude list. The more I focused on positive thoughts and the many blessings I have, the better I felt!

Now it's your turn to do the same. I believe you can make the changes you desire to make, but it will take effort. It will take time on your part. It will take planning and preparation for you to be successful. You will need to think hard about why you want to make the necessary changes.

There's no time for us to make excuses. We need to be bold and courageous. We need to trust in our God. We need to fill our minds with positive thoughts. Remember what the apostle Paul said in **Philippians 4:8**:

"Finally, brothers, whatever is true, whatever is honorable, whatever is just, whatever is pure, whatever is lovely, whatever is commendable, if there

Cover design © 2017 by Edify Media
Interior Design © 2017 by Edify Media
Contact Edify Media at Facebook.com/EdifyMediaMDW

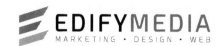

is any excellence, if there is anything worthy of praise, think about these things."

The Holy Spirit reminds us about the power of our mind and our thoughts. Christians' minds should be focused on our Jesus. When we allow junk into our minds, bad things will happen. Our minds are powerful. We need to be careful how think. The same could be said with respect to how we talk to ourselves. Many people speak to themselves in a way they would never speak to others. When people constantly tell themselves, "I stink," "I'm worthless," or "I'm never going to be successful" they become what they tell themselves. Be careful how you speak to yourself. Be careful with what you allow into your mind. Our brains are powerful! We are reminded in Psalm 139:14,

"...I am fearfully and wonderfully made..."

When I began my journey in 2016, I visualized myself being successful. Now I want you to do the same. This journal will help you to grow in your faith, enjoy the blessings God has given you, and accomplish your fitness goals.

This journal is designed to guide you through the first 31 days of your transformation. It also can be at any point in your transformation.

Everyday, you have space to...
- Write out your daily prayer to God. We need time to pray, Mark 1:35.
- Write out five things you are grateful for each day. We have many reasons to overflow with gratitude, Colossians 2:7.
- What kind of exercise you will perform for the day.
- What you plan to eat and then what you actually ate. This will help you in future planning to see where you can improve.
- A space to write out something motivational for yourself.
- You will also be able to read a motivational thought from me to help you along the way.

I'm excited about the great changes you are about to make. Now I just have one question for you? **Are you ready?**

Don't waste a day...
Don't waste an hour...
Don't waste a minute...
Don't waste a second...
Don't waste any of your workouts.
You will regret you did.

You get a choice...live and learn OR learn and live....

Now is the time for us to grow in all aspects of our lives. Now is your TIME. Go get it. Don't wait until TOMORROW. Don't wait until the next MONDAY. And remember that SOMEDAY is not a day of the WEEK! Today is the DAY you start.

– Benjamin Lee
Follow Benjamin at benjaminleeonline.com and benjaminlee.blog.

DAY 1

BE HAPPY IN YOUR SHOES

There's someone right now who would love to be in your shoes! There is someone who would love to be able to put on those workout clothes, sit in traffic, endure the cold weather, and wake up early to go to the gym to workout.

They would love to feel sweaty. They would love to feel their bodies getting stronger. They would love to stand upright and flex in the mirror. They would love to experience the feeling of running, of doing push ups, or gripping weights.

Don't take for granted what you can do. There are many who would love to have weights in their house! Take nothing for granted! Get up, fight, work, sweat, rejoice and no complaining! Take nothing for granted!

Yeah, I'm talking to you!!! Get Up!

FAITH: Write out your prayers to God.

_____

_____

_____

_____

_____

_____

_____

_____

FITNESS: What's your game plan today?

For my body, today I will...

_____

_____

_____

Exercise Your Mind

Write out "I am successful."

_____

_____

FAMILY: Make a gratitude list.

1. _____

2. _____

3. _____

4. _____

5. _____

FOOD: What are you planning to eat?

1. _____

2. _____

3. _____

4. _____

5. _____

6. _____

What did you actually eat?

1. _____

2. _____

3. _____

4. _____

5. _____

6. _____

Celebrate what you did right today
with your eating.

DAY 2

EMBRACE THE CHALLENGE

Embrace the challenge! Whether it's the holiday season or the middle of June, you need to do the impossible, or at least the impossible in the eyes of many. You need to stay on track. Who cares if it is the holiday season. Who cares if you are on vacation. Who cares if you are busy. You must find a way.

Life is a challenge, so go ahead and embrace it. Eating healthy while travelling is a challenge. Eating healthy while taking care of children is a challenge. Embrace the challenge. Eating healthy and working out even when you don't want to is a challenge. Embrace the challenge and crush it.

You are going to eat healthy! You are going to lose weight and build muscle! You are going to change your body for life. This must become an obsession! Think about it, breathe it, live it, crush it.

Yeah, I'm talking to you!!! Get up!!!

FAITH: Write out your prayers to God.

_____

_____

_____

_____

_____

_____

_____

_____

FITNESS: What's your game plan today?

For my body, today I will...

_____

_____

_____

Exercise Your Mind

Write out "I am successful."

_____

_____

FAMILY: Make a gratitude list.

1. _____

2. _____

3. _____

4. _____

5. _____

FOOD: What are you planning to eat?

1. _____

2. _____

3. _____

4. _____

5. _____

6. _____

What did you actually eat?

1. _____

2. _____

3. _____

4. _____

5. _____

6. _____

Celebrate what you did right today
with your eating.

DAY **3**

IT'S TIME

It's time for work!
It's time for change!
It's time for strength!
It's time to flourish!
It's time for explosive change!
It's time, baby! It's time, baby!
It's time to break through!

Yeah, I'm talking to you!!! Get up!!!

FAITH: Write out your prayers to God.

_____

_____

_____

_____

_____

_____

_____

_____

FITNESS: What's your game plan today?

For my body, today I will...

_____

_____

_____

Exercise Your Mind

Write out "I am successful."

_____

_____

FAMILY: Make a gratitude list.

1. _____

2. _____

3. _____

4. _____

5. _____

FOOD: What are you planning to eat?

1. _____

2. _____

3. _____

4. _____

5. _____

6. _____

What did you actually eat?

1. _____

2. _____

3. _____

4. _____

5. _____

6. _____

Celebrate what you did right today with your eating.

DAY 4

CHANGE

Transformation is about change. You can't remain the same. You must push forward, and leave the past in the past. Remember, every day is another opportunity for you to change. But you must decide you are ready to pay the price it will take to change. The sacrifice will be worth it.

Yeah, I'm talking to you!!! Get up!!!

FAITH: Write out your prayers to God.

_____

_____

_____

_____

_____

_____

_____

_____

FITNESS: What's your game plan today?

For my body, today I will...

_____

_____

_____

Exercise Your Mind

Write out "I am successful."

_____

_____

FAMILY: Make a gratitude list.

1. _____

2. _____

3. _____

4. _____

5. _____

FOOD: What are you planning to eat?

1. _____

2. _____

3. _____

4. _____

5. _____

6. _____

What did you actually eat?

1. _____

2. _____

3. _____

4. _____

5. _____

6. _____

Celebrate what you did right today with your eating.

DAY 5
DO IT AGAIN

You're on Day 5, and you are doing a great job! Keep it going. Don't give up. Get up and go exercise. Motivate yourself, and remember your goals.

Yeah, I'm talking to you!!! Get up!!!

FAITH: Write out your prayers to God.

_____

_____

_____

_____

_____

_____

_____

_____

FITNESS: What's your game plan today?

For my body, today I will...

_____

_____

_____

Exercise Your Mind

Write out "I am successful."

_____

_____

FAMILY: Make a gratitude list.

1. _____

2. _____

3. _____

4. _____

5. _____

FOOD: What are you planning to eat?

1. _____

2. _____

3. _____

4. _____

5. _____

6. _____

What did you actually eat?

1. _____

2. _____

3. _____

4. _____

5. _____

6. _____

Celebrate what you did right today
with your eating.

DAY 6

NO MORE SELF SABOTAGE

Get out of your own way, and be victorious. Allow yourself to be successful. Don't be afraid to accomplish your goals. Go get them!!! Right now!

It's time to crank it out like never before. There can be no excuses. It doesn't matter if you have to travel a lot. That's not an excuse for you to sabotage your efforts. Failure is not an option. There are people who need you to be strong.

Every day you decide to make a change, you will become stronger. Don't be afraid of success. Don't sabotage all of your hard work. Keep going.

Yeah, I'm talking to you!!! Get up!!!

FAITH: Write out your prayers to God.

_____

_____

_____

_____

_____

_____

_____

_____

FITNESS: What's your game plan today?

For my body, today I will...

_____

_____

_____

Exercise Your Mind

Write out "I am successful."

_____

_____

_____

FAMILY: Make a gratitude list.

1. _____

2. _____

3. _____

4. _____

5. _____

FOOD: What are you planning to eat?

1. _____

2. _____

3. _____

4. _____

5. _____

6. _____

What did you actually eat?

1. _____

2. _____

3. _____

4. _____

5. _____

6. _____

Celebrate what you did right today
with your eating.

DAY 7

DON'T WAIT FOR ANYONE

Don't wait for anybody...Just Go!!!
Sometimes, you can't wait...
You can't wait for your spouse to get on board!
You can't wait for your children to have 100% buy in...
You just have to GO!!!
Go and push for those goals.
Go and workout...
Go and encourage others...
Go, Go, Go....
Sometimes, you can't wait.
Waiting on your spouse to change may mean that you never change.
Instead, you will have to be the change. You can't wait for the perfect conditions...
You can't wait for the perfect time of year...
You have to do it right now!!!!
Get up right now and be the change!
Be the ambassador in your house.
Even if you haven't arrived to where you want to be, act like you are there. Your body will soon catch up with your mind...
Can you hear me? Go, right now!!!
Others will catch up with you later.

Yeah, I'm talking to you!!! Get up!!!

FAITH: Write out your prayers to God.

_____

_____

_____

_____

_____

_____

_____

_____

FITNESS: What's your game plan today?

For my body, today I will...

_____

_____

_____

Exercise Your Mind

Write out "I am successful."

_____

_____

_____

FAMILY: Make a gratitude list.

1. _____

2. _____

3. _____

4. _____

5. _____

FOOD: What are you planning to eat?

1. _____

2. _____

3. _____

4. _____

5. _____

6. _____

What did you actually eat?

1. _____

2. _____

3. _____

4. _____

5. _____

6. _____

Celebrate what you did right today
with your eating.

DAY 8

PAY THE FEE

If you want to get something, you will have to pay the fee. You will have to say "No" to get to your "Yes."

Get up and pay the cost!
The cost of greatness!
The cost of accomplishing your goals!
The cost of getting to the mountain top!
The cost of living the dream!
Pay it right now!
Pay it every day!
Cmon!! Let out that scream at the gym, on the bike path, in your basement, or wherever you workout!
Pay the cost for excellence! And enjoy every cent of it!

Yeah, I'm talking to you!!! Get up!!!

FAITH: Write out your prayers to God.

_____

_____

_____

_____

_____

_____

_____

_____

FITNESS: What's your game plan today?

For my body, today I will...

_____

_____

_____

Exercise Your Mind

Write out "I am successful."

_____

_____

FAMILY: Make a gratitude list.

1. _____

2. _____

3. _____

4. _____

5. _____

FOOD: What are you planning to eat?

1. _____

2. _____

3. _____

4. _____

5. _____

6. _____

What did you actually eat?

1. _____

2. _____

3. _____

4. _____

5. _____

6. _____

Celebrate what you did right today with your eating.

DAY 9

FIND MORE LEVERAGE

Find more leverage....

I found some more leverage in my closet!
A suit I haven't worn in a really long time! I was thinking, "I wonder if it fits?" It does! How clothes fit don't lie. Neither does the mirror.

Find what you need to stay focused! Is it that holiday party? That dress? That suit? Is it your children? What can you find today that will help you to stay on track? Whatever it is, use it.

Yeah, I'm talking to you!!! Get Up!!!

FAITH: Write out your prayers to God.

_____

_____

_____

_____

_____

_____

_____

FITNESS: What's your game plan today?

For my body, today I will...

_____

_____

_____

Exercise Your Mind

Write out "I am successful."

_____

_____

FAMILY: Make a gratitude list.

1. _____

2. _____

3. _____

4. _____

5. _____

FOOD: What are you planning to eat?

1. _____

2. _____

3. _____

4. _____

5. _____

6. _____

What did you actually eat?

1. _____

2. _____

3. _____

4. _____

5. _____

6. _____

Celebrate what you did right today with your eating.

DAY 10

I'M NOT GOING BACK

Don't go back!

No more before photos! Push it! Do more!
Make sure you don't go back! Don't go back to
being lazy, wishing but never taking action. Don't
quit. Remember what you told yourself you would
do back on Day 1. Be sure to keep the commitment
you made.

Yeah, I'm talking to you! Get Up!!!

FAITH: Write out your prayers to God.

_____

_____

_____

_____

_____

_____

_____

_____

FITNESS: What's your game plan today?

For my body, today I will...

_____

_____

_____

Exercise Your Mind

Write out "I am successful."

_____

_____

_____

FAMILY: Make a gratitude list.

1. _____

2. _____

3. _____

4. _____

5. _____

FOOD: What are you planning to eat?

1. _____

2. _____

3. _____

4. _____

5. _____

6. _____

What did you actually eat?

1. _____

2. _____

3. _____

4. _____

5. _____

6. _____

Celebrate what you did right today with your eating.

DAY 11

CONTROL WHAT YOU CAN CONTROL

It's time to take it up another notch!
You only can control what you can control! But you can control a lot.

I can't control genetics and an enlarged heart. I couldn't control the blood clot in my heart that decided to show up while I was on the treadmill two years ago. But I can control my attitude. I can control my eating consumption. I can control making the most of my time.

There are so many things out of our control. But let's not use that as an excuse for not controlling what you can control!

What feels good? The compliments, the feeling of great health, keeping your commitment, accomplishing those goals? Hold on to positive thoughts as people try to suck you back to your former self. Your former self is gone!!! Don't bring him/her back. Keep him/her buried! Someone scream with me...Go, go, go!!!

Yeah, I'm talking to you!!! Get Up!!!

FAITH: Write out your prayers to God.

_____

_____

_____

_____

_____

_____

_____

FITNESS: What's your game plan today?

For my body, today I will...

_____

_____

_____

Exercise Your Mind

Write out "I am successful."

_____

_____

FAMILY: Make a gratitude list.

1. _____

2. _____

3. _____

4. _____

5. _____

FOOD: What are you planning to eat?

1. _____

2. _____

3. _____

4. _____

5. _____

6. _____

What did you actually eat?

1. _____

2. _____

3. _____

4. _____

5. _____

6. _____

Celebrate what you did right today
with your eating.

DAY **12**

I CAN, I WILL, I AM

Transforming and making real changes requires you to keep a positive mindset. During this process, you will have to talk to yourself positively. That's part of motivating yourself.

Remind yourself you can, you will, and you are successful right now.

Yeah, I'm talking to you!!! Let's Go!!!

FAITH: Write out your prayers to God.

_____

_____

_____

_____

_____

_____

_____

FITNESS: What's your game plan today?

For my body, today I will...

_____

_____

_____

Exercise Your Mind

Write out "I am successful."

_____

_____

FAMILY: Make a gratitude list.

1. _____

2. _____

3. _____

4. _____

5. _____

FOOD: What are you planning to eat?

1. _____

2. _____

3. _____

4. _____

5. _____

6. _____

What did you actually eat?

1. _____

2. _____

3. _____

4. _____

5. _____

6. _____

Celebrate what you did right today
with your eating.

DAY 13

FIND A WAY

There will be times when life will be challenging. Life happens! But somehow you are going to have to find a way. This may require you to wake up earlier than normal. Or you may need to stay up later than usual, so you can get in that workout. When life gets busy, you might get a little too relaxed with exercise and your time with God. You can't allow that to happen. Find a way.

Yeah, I'm talking to you!!! Get Up!!!

FAITH: Write out your prayers to God.

_____

_____

_____

_____

_____

_____

_____

FITNESS: What's your game plan today?

For my body, today I will...

_____

_____

_____

Exercise Your Mind

Write out "I am successful."

_____

_____

_____

FAMILY: Make a gratitude list.

1. _____

2. _____

3. _____

4. _____

5. _____

FOOD: What are you planning to eat?

1. _____

2. _____

3. _____

4. _____

5. _____

6. _____

What did you actually eat?

1. _____

2. _____

3. _____

4. _____

5. _____

6. _____

Celebrate what you did right today
with your eating.

DAY 14

THE FOOD IS NOT GOING ANYWHERE

Let's face, you know how to eat! Sometimes you can eat like there will not be a tomorrow. But breathe, and take a step back from that cookie or cinnamon roll. Do you really need to eat that? Don't worry, you can say "NO" now, so you can say "YES" later. The food is not going anywhere. Stay on track.

Yeah, I'm talking to you!!! Get Up!!!

FAITH: Write out your prayers to God.

_____

_____

_____

_____

_____

_____

_____

_____

FITNESS: What's your game plan today?

For my body, today I will...

_____

_____

_____

Exercise Your Mind

Write out "I am successful."

_____

_____

FAMILY: Make a gratitude list.

1. _____

2. _____

3. _____

4. _____

5. _____

FOOD: What are you planning to eat?

1. _____

2. _____

3. _____

4. _____

5. _____

6. _____

What did you actually eat?

1. _____

2. _____

3. _____

4. _____

5. _____

6. _____

Celebrate what you did right today with your eating.

DAY 15

PEOPLE ARE WATCHING YOU

This journey to better health and a better life is not merely about you. There are people watching you right now. Yes, that's right. It could be your spouse.

Or maybe your children. For some, it could be some-one at work. Here's the point. By staying the course, you have no idea how you may be able to assist someone later in life. But if you give up now, you'll never know what could have been. Cmon!

Yeah, I'm talking to you!!! Get Up!!!

FAITH: Write out your prayers to God.

_____

_____

_____

_____

_____

_____

_____

_____

FITNESS: What's your game plan today?

For my body, today I will...

_____

_____

_____

Exercise Your Mind

Write out "I am successful."

_____

_____

FAMILY: Make a gratitude list.

1. _____

2. _____

3. _____

4. _____

5. _____

FOOD: What are you planning to eat?

1. _____

2. _____

3. _____

4. _____

5. _____

6. _____

What did you actually eat?

1. _____

2. _____

3. _____

4. _____

5. _____

6. _____

Celebrate what you did right today
with your eating.

DAY 16

I WILL

I will honor my promises.
I will transform for LIFE.
I will keep my commitments to God.
I will keep my commitments to my family.
I WILL...Go ahead and say it with me... "I WILL SUCCEED."

Yeah, I'm talking to you!!! Get Up!!!

FAITH: Write out your prayers to God.

_____

_____

_____

_____

_____

_____

_____

_____

FAMILY: Make a gratitude list.

1. _____

2. _____

3. _____

4. _____

5. _____

FOOD: What are you planning to eat?

1. _____

2. _____

3. _____

4. _____

5. _____

6. _____

FITNESS: What's your game plan today?

For my body, today I will...

_____

_____

_____

What did you actually eat?

1. _____

2. _____

3. _____

4. _____

5. _____

6. _____

Exercise Your Mind

Write out "I am successful."

_____

_____

_____

Celebrate what you did right today with your eating.

DAY 17

YOUR ONE CHANCE

I didn't want to look back when I was a 40 year old man and say, "Man, I should have entered that preaching training program in Beaumont, TX."

So, I decided to move across country with my wife into the unknown! It was an Abraham-moment. I was 30 and recently out of a job with Pfizer. I kept my job during downsizing in 2006, but not in 2009. After eight years, it was time for something new. I had been thinking about preaching for a long time. I could have found another sales job. But the timing seemed right. There was a great need (and still is) for preachers (who are willing to work).

Life is about taking risks, right? I didn't want to look back with regret! This may be my one chance! I'm glad I took that chance. Why am I saying all of this? Maybe this is your MOMENT! Maybe this is your FINAL CHANCE!!! "Your only chance" kind of moment.

What if this your One Chance? Will you take advantage of it? Did you push (really push) yourself in those workouts? What if this is the One Time, the Right Time, the Last Time moment for you to make the changes you've been dreaming about for months, years? Leave nothing on the table!

The time is now folks! Go get it!

Yeah, I'm talking to you!!! Get Up!!!

FAITH: Write out your prayers to God.

_____

_____

_____

_____

_____

_____

_____

_____

FITNESS: What's your game plan today?

For my body, today I will...

_____

_____

_____

Exercise Your Mind

Write out "I am successful."

_____

_____

FAMILY: Make a gratitude list.

1. _____

2. _____

3. _____

4. _____

5. _____

FOOD: What are you planning to eat?

1. _____

2. _____

3. _____

4. _____

5. _____

6. _____

What did you actually eat?

1. _____

2. _____

3. _____

4. _____

5. _____

6. _____

Celebrate what you did right today
with your eating.

DAY 18

BLESSED BEYOND MEASURE

Do you realize how blessed you really are? Has the gratitude list been helping you? Indeed, you are so blessed. The fact that you have life and the ability to exercise is reason for you to be thankful. Don't take for granted the opportunities you have right in front of you.

Yeah, I'm talking to you!!! Get Up!!!

FAITH: Write out your prayers to God.

_____

_____

_____

_____

_____

_____

_____

_____

FITNESS: What's your game plan today?

For my body, today I will...

_____

_____

_____

Exercise Your Mind

Write out "I am successful."

_____

_____

FAMILY: Make a gratitude list.

1. _____

2. _____

3. _____

4. _____

5. _____

FOOD: What are you planning to eat?

1. _____

2. _____

3. _____

4. _____

5. _____

6. _____

What did you actually eat?

1. _____

2. _____

3. _____

4. _____

5. _____

6. _____

Celebrate what you did right today with your eating.

DAY 19

DON'T DROP THE BALL
ON THE ONE-YARD LINE

Am I the only one who has screamed at the television when watching football, "What are you doing?" While I haven't watched any games so far this year, I've seen the highlights. In particular, I've seen the replays of players on the verge of scoring only to drop the ball at the ONE YARD LINE!!!!!

Have they lost their minds? They don't follow through all the way! As a result, instead of winning, they will often find themselves losing! Don't drop the ball at the ONE YARD LINE! You are on the verge of great success! You are getting closer to the end zone! Make sure you don't drop the ball at the ONE LINE YARD LINE!

You must follow through with your meal preparation.

You must follow through with your exercise regimen.

You can't allow a heavy workload to cause you to fumble!

You can't allow rocky relationships to cause you to fumble. You can't control others, but you can control our emotional state, how you respond, what you eat, and your intensity with your workouts. Don't fumble at the one.

There's only one opponent in your game! It's the person you see in the mirror every day. It's overcoming those self-limiting beliefs. It's keeping those commitments you've made to yourself. It's about investing in the future.

These players fumble at the ONE YARD LINE fumble because of themselves. No one else causes them to fumble. They defeat themselves. You would think they would learn from all the other players who have done it before them not to make the same mistake. But they don't. What about you?

You know what works! You know those who have been successful have stuck to the plan. Do the same. Don't become your own worst enemy. Don't fumble at the ONE YARD LINE!

Yeah, I'm talking to you!!! Get Up!!!

FAITH: Write out your prayers to God.

_____

_____

_____

_____

_____

_____

_____

_____

FITNESS: What's your game plan today?

For my body, today I will...

_____

_____

_____

Exercise Your Mind

Write out "I am successful."

_____

_____

FAMILY: Make a gratitude list.

1. _____

2. _____

3. _____

4. _____

5. _____

FOOD: What are you planning to eat?

1. _____

2. _____

3. _____

4. _____

5. _____

6. _____

What did you actually eat?

1. _____

2. _____

3. _____

4. _____

5. _____

6. _____

Celebrate what you did right today with your eating.

DAY 20
THE NO EXCUSE ZONE

DATE_____

You are in the no excuse zone. All excuses have to be put to the side.

Even if you are driving across country there are no excuses. Get in your workout. You can eat well and exercise.

Even if you are in the armed services, there are no excuses. You can eat well and exercise.

Even if you are working 12 hours a day, there are no excuses. You can still eat well and exercise.

Even if you are a stay-at-home mom, busy with the children, there are no excuses. You can still eat well and exercise.

Even if you travel a lot for your job, there are no excuses. You can still eat well and exercise.

Even if you travel outside of the U.S., there are no excuses. You can still eat well and exercise.

Even if you are physically injured, there are no excuses You can still eat well and do mental exercises.

There are no excuses! Do you want this? How far are you willing to go to accomplish your goal? Will you go to bed a little bit earlier? Will you wake up a little earlier? Will you focus on complaining less (even better, not at all)?

Yeah, I'm talking to you!!! Get Up!!!

FAITH: Write out your prayers to God.

_____

_____

_____

_____

_____

_____

_____

_____

FAMILY: Make a gratitude list.

1. _____

2. _____

3. _____

4. _____

5. _____

FOOD: What are you planning to eat?

1. _____

2. _____

3. _____

4. _____

5. _____

6. _____

FITNESS: What's your game plan today?

For my body, today I will...

_____

_____

_____

What did you actually eat?

1. _____

2. _____

3. _____

4. _____

5. _____

6. _____

Exercise Your Mind

Write out "I am successful."

_____

_____

Celebrate what you did right today with your eating.

FAITH: Write out your prayers to God.

_____

DAY 21

DATE_____

DON'T FOCUS ON WHAT'S WRONG; FOCUS ON WHAT'S RIGHT

It's easy to zoom in on everything that is wrong...

You may not like your job
You may not like your house
You may not like your spouse (oh, boy!)
You may not like your finances
You may not like your body

Focusing on what's wrong accomplishes nothing! Oh wait, yes it does! It produces unhappiness, unmet goals, and a vicious, toxic cycle that only brings pain and not pleasure.

Focus on what's right!

You have a job
You have a house
You have a spouse (a lot of singles would love to have marital problems).
You have some money
You still have a body that works

Focus on the positives! Overflow with gratitude!

You're taking control of your health! You have hope! Your bodies will change! That's the easy part! Changing our minds is where the real transformation occurs!

As you go to work, appreciate your job.
Appreciate the shelter you do have!
Give your spouse a big kiss on the way out the door!
Really appreciate that you are taking charge of your health!

Yeah, I'm talking to you!!! Get Up!!!

FAITH: Write out your prayers to God.

_____

_____

_____

_____

_____

_____

_____

FAMILY: Make a gratitude list.

1. _____

2. _____

3. _____

4. _____

5. _____

FOOD: What are you planning to eat?

1. _____

2. _____

3. _____

4. _____

5. _____

6. _____

FITNESS: What's your game plan today?

For my body, today I will...

_____

_____

_____

What did you actually eat?

1. _____

2. _____

3. _____

4. _____

5. _____

6. _____

Exercise Your Mind

Write out "I am successful."

_____

_____

Celebrate what you did right today with your eating.

DAY 22

JOIN THE CLUB!!!

Tuesday afternoon...about 3:13 p.m...2014. I'm at 6mph on the treadmill, warming up. I'm about 5 minutes in when I feel "it." What's the "it?" I'm not quite sure. But "it" is making all my teeth hurt! "It" is making me sweat like crazy. "It" is making me feel extremely tired!

"It" forces me stop the treadmill and ask myself the question "is this 'it' a heart attack? I'm 36. I'm too young to have a heart attack. I just helped someone move a few hours ago. I'm supposed to be recording a broadcast later today, so this can't be happening."

"It" eventually forces me to leave the gym and make my way to the hospital, where I'm told that I'm having a heart attack! What! No way!

The next day, I get some additional information about "it." The arteries in my heart are clean as a whistle! "It" was a blood clot in my right coronary artery! Wow! "It" rearranges my entire life and thoughts! I'm at a rehab with a 70 year old doing a top speed of 1.9mph on the treadmill. Noooooo!!!! I'm depressed, angry, and confused. Thankfully, "it" doesn't define me and what I can do. I had people that helped me. I would get back on that same treadmill at the same time a year later and do about 5 miles. I still have a ways to go but the fear is gone.

What's your "it?" We all have one. Will it define you? Will it cause you to quit?

Join the club!

We all have an "it". Before you throw a pity party, remember everyone has an "it." Use that "it" to grow, not to die! Use it to push yourself, not to quit! Use it to push others rather to isolate others!

Join the club and prosper!

Yeah, I'm talking to you!!! Get Up!!!

FAITH: Write out your prayers to God.

_____

_____

_____

_____

_____

_____

_____

_____

FITNESS: What's your game plan today?

For my body, today I will...

_____

_____

_____

Exercise Your Mind

Write out "I am successful."

_____

_____

_____

FAMILY: Make a gratitude list.

1. _____

2. _____

3. _____

4. _____

5. _____

FOOD: What are you planning to eat?

1. _____

2. _____

3. _____

4. _____

5. _____

6. _____

What did you actually eat?

1. _____

2. _____

3. _____

4. _____

5. _____

6. _____

Celebrate what you did right today
with your eating.

DAY 23

THERE CAN BE NO QUIT

There can be no quit.
Go get the real you! Go get her.
You know the one I'm talking about!
She's in there! She's waiting for you to say "no more,
I refuse to be defeated! I can't be stopped! Let's go!"

Go get the real you! Go get him.
You know the one I'm talking about!
The man who is strong and confident. He is in there,
waiting to come out.
Did you work out? Cmon! There can be no quit!!

Yeah, I'm talking to you!!! Get Up!!!

FAITH: Write out your prayers to God.

_____

_____

_____

_____

_____

_____

_____

_____

FITNESS: What's your game plan today?

For my body, today I will...

_____

_____

_____

Exercise Your Mind

Write out "I am successful."

_____

_____

FAMILY: Make a gratitude list.

1. _____

2. _____

3. _____

4. _____

5. _____

FOOD: What are you planning to eat?

1. _____

2. _____

3. _____

4. _____

5. _____

6. _____

What did you actually eat?

1. _____

2. _____

3. _____

4. _____

5. _____

6. _____

Celebrate what you did right today
with your eating.

DAY 24

YOU ARE DOING SO WELL

Wow, it's already been 24 days. Can you believe how fast time flies when you're having fun? Let's keep it going. Give yourself a pat on the back. Continue to look forward, and take time to appreciate what you have accomplished.

Yeah, I'm talking to you!! Get Up!

FAITH: Write out your prayers to God.

_____

_____

_____

_____

_____

_____

_____

_____

FITNESS: What's your game plan today?

For my body, today I will...

_____

_____

_____

Exercise Your Mind

Write out "I am successful."

_____

_____

FAMILY: Make a gratitude list.

1. _____

2. _____

3. _____

4. _____

5. _____

FOOD: What are you planning to eat?

1. _____

2. _____

3. _____

4. _____

5. _____

6. _____

What did you actually eat?

1. _____

2. _____

3. _____

4. _____

5. _____

6. _____

Celebrate what you did right today
with your eating.

DAY 25

WHAT IF

What if you worked out as much as you watched television?

What if you worked out as much as you scrolled through Facebook? What if you worked out as much as you complained? What if?

What if you harnessed your energy for good and changed your body and your life? It doesn't have to be a "what if" scenario. It can be an " I CAN DO and I WILL DO" moment.

Yeah, I'm talking to you!!! Get Up!!!

FAITH: Write out your prayers to God.

_____

_____

_____

_____

_____

_____

_____

_____

FITNESS: What's your game plan today?

For my body, today I will...

_____

_____

_____

Exercise Your Mind

Write out "I am successful."

_____

_____

FAMILY: Make a gratitude list.

1. _____

2. _____

3. _____

4. _____

5. _____

FOOD: What are you planning to eat?

1. _____

2. _____

3. _____

4. _____

5. _____

6. _____

What did you actually eat?

1. _____

2. _____

3. _____

4. _____

5. _____

6. _____

Celebrate what you did right today
with your eating.

DAY 26
NO MORE

No more quick fixes....
No more weird diets...
Your problem likely is that you have been lazy and have overeaten for a long time. Carbs are not the problem, and sugar is not the problem. Overeating and laziness are problems.

It's time to move! It's time to eat healthy with the proper foods and portions....
It's time!! Are you ready? Or are you going to use more excuses to overeat and kill your body?

Yeah, I'm talking to you!!! Get up!!!!

FAITH: Write out your prayers to God.

_____

_____

_____

_____

_____

_____

_____

_____

FITNESS: What's your game plan today?

For my body, today I will...

_____

_____

_____

Exercise Your Mind

Write out "I am successful."

_____

_____

FAMILY: Make a gratitude list.

1. _____

2. _____

3. _____

4. _____

5. _____

FOOD: What are you planning to eat?

1. _____

2. _____

3. _____

4. _____

5. _____

6. _____

What did you actually eat?

1. _____

2. _____

3. _____

4. _____

5. _____

6. _____

Celebrate what you did right today
with your eating.

DAY 27

IT'S A NEW DAY

It's a new day!
A day of new opportunities!
A day to draw closer to God.
A day to draw closer and to trust Him even more.
A day of worship.
A day of planning.
A new day!
Enjoy, and make the most of it.

Yeah, I'm talking to you!!! Get Up!!!

FAITH: Write out your prayers to God.

_____

_____

_____

_____

_____

_____

_____

_____

FITNESS: What's your game plan today?

For my body, today I will...

_____

_____

_____

Exercise Your Mind

Write out "I am successful."

_____

_____

FAMILY: Make a gratitude list.

1. _____

2. _____

3. _____

4. _____

5. _____

FOOD: What are you planning to eat?

1. _____

2. _____

3. _____

4. _____

5. _____

6. _____

What did you actually eat?

1. _____

2. _____

3. _____

4. _____

5. _____

6. _____

Celebrate what you did right today with your eating.

DAY 28

THERE CAN BE NO GOING BACK

Tired of losing the same weight over and over? Not doing it anymore. How much weight have you lost? 100 pounds? Some would say, "no way." But if you're losing the same 20 pounds every two years over a decade that's 100 pounds. Cmon! Are you fed up yet? Change your language. Instead of "losing weight" how about releasing the weight once and for all.

Yeah, I'm talking to you!!! Get Up!!!

FAITH: Write out your prayers to God.

_____

_____

_____

_____

_____

_____

_____

_____

FITNESS: What's your game plan today?

For my body, today I will...

_____

_____

_____

Exercise Your Mind

Write out "I am successful."

_____

_____

FAMILY: Make a gratitude list.

1. _____

2. _____

3. _____

4. _____

5. _____

FOOD: What are you planning to eat?

1. _____

2. _____

3. _____

4. _____

5. _____

6. _____

What did you actually eat?

1. _____

2. _____

3. _____

4. _____

5. _____

6. _____

Celebrate what you did right today
with your eating.

DAY **29**

IT'S NOT MAGIC, SILLY

The waistline won't shrink on its own. The muscles won't develop overnight. You must put in the work. So go do it now!

Yeah, I'm talking to you!!! Get Up!!!

FAITH: Write out your prayers to God.

_____

_____

_____

_____

_____

_____

_____

FITNESS: What's your game plan today?

For my body, today I will...

_____

_____

_____

Exercise Your Mind

Write out "I am successful."

_____

_____

FAMILY: Make a gratitude list.

1. _____

2. _____

3. _____

4. _____

5. _____

FOOD: What are you planning to eat?

1. _____

2. _____

3. _____

4. _____

5. _____

6. _____

What did you actually eat?

1. _____

2. _____

3. _____

4. _____

5. _____

6. _____

Celebrate what you did right today
with your eating.

DAY 30

WHEN LIFE HITS

When adversity hits you in the gut...

When stressful times come rolling in like a thunderstorm...

When disappointment moves into your house and doesn't seem to leave...

Be sure you turn to God. Stay connected with Him...

And be sure to exercise...

Exercise is one of the great anti-depressants!

When I graduated from college in 2001, and was looking for a job, I made sure to exercise.

When I got a job promotion in 2006, I made sure I was exercising. That was a stressful moment.

When I got released in 2009 due to cuts, I made sure I was exercising.

When my dad was going through chemo, I made sure i was exercising.

When Dad died, and I had to preach his funeral, I made sure I exercised. That was a tough day, week, month, year.

When my grandparents died, and I preached their funerals, I made sure I was exercising.

When Nikki and I experienced a molar pregnancy and tremendous disappointment, I did my best to exercise.

As I looked at my wife curled up on the couch, exhausted and frustrated, I tried my best to exercise.

When I got a blood clot in my heart, I was actually exercising. I made sure to get back to exercising (1.7 mph) on treadmill (better something than nothing).

After getting two defibrillators, I made sure (and am making sure) I'm exercising.

My point? Each of us will experience an "IT" something that wants to defeat us, crush us, destroy us!

What's your IT? How will you respond? Turn to God! Rely on Him. Release your anger, fear, and disappointment in a positive way. You could turn to FOOD. You will feel good for a moment and then have guilt and fat afterwards.

Fight back! Move. Get up! Never give up!

Yeah I'm talking to you! Get Up!!!

FAITH: Write out your prayers to God.

_____

_____

_____

_____

_____

_____

_____

_____

FITNESS: What's your game plan today?

For my body, today I will...

_____

_____

_____

Exercise Your Mind

Write out "I am successful."

_____

_____

FAMILY: Make a gratitude list.

1. _____

2. _____

3. _____

4. _____

5. _____

FOOD: What are you planning to eat?

1. _____

2. _____

3. _____

4. _____

5. _____

6. _____

What did you actually eat?

1. _____

2. _____

3. _____

4. _____

5. _____

6. _____

Celebrate what you did right today
with your eating.

DAY 31

IT DOESN'T MATTER

Rain or shine
Sleep or no sleep
Stressed or relaxed
Busy or bored
Hungry or full
Crying or laughing
Day or night
Employed or unemployed
Get your workout in...
If you can walk, then walk, if you can run then run, if you can lift them lift!
C'mon now! Yeah I'm talking to you!
There's no turning back!

Yeah, I'm talking to you!!! Get Up!!!

FAITH: Write out your prayers to God.

_____

_____

_____

_____

_____

_____

_____

_____

FITNESS: What's your game plan today?

For my body, today I will...

_____

_____

_____

Exercise Your Mind

Write out "I am successful."

_____

_____

FAMILY: Make a gratitude list.

1. _____

2. _____

3. _____

4. _____

5. _____

FOOD: What are you planning to eat?

1. _____

2. _____

3. _____

4. _____

5. _____

6. _____

What did you actually eat?

1. _____

2. _____

3. _____

4. _____

5. _____

6. _____

Celebrate what you did right today
with your eating.

— YES! YES! YES! —

You've made it through an entire month. You have focused and worked hard on your body, your mind-set, and hopefully your walk with God. How are you doing? How are you feeling?

There's no turning back now! Keep it going and stay focused. This journal is designed to propel you to continue to journal. Every day motivate yourself, be thankful, and talk to God.

Everyday we get a choice. We can either choose to do the right things or the wrong things. The choice is ours. What will you do? Where will you turn? No more wasting time! Get the job done. Work harder and do more. You will be successful. You will win. Finish the job my friend!

– Benjamin Lee
Follow Benjamin at benjaminleeonline.com
and benjaminlee.blog.

Made in the USA
San Bernardino, CA
27 September 2017